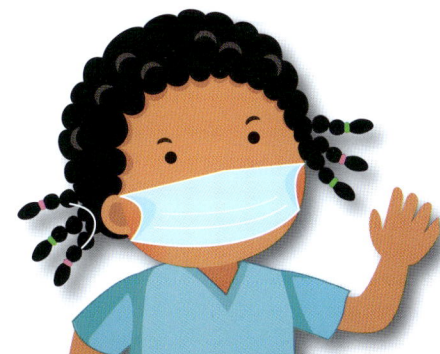
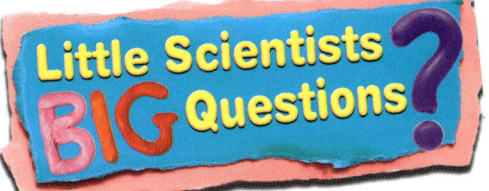

How Does a Dentist Use Science?

Written and Designed by **Alix Wood**

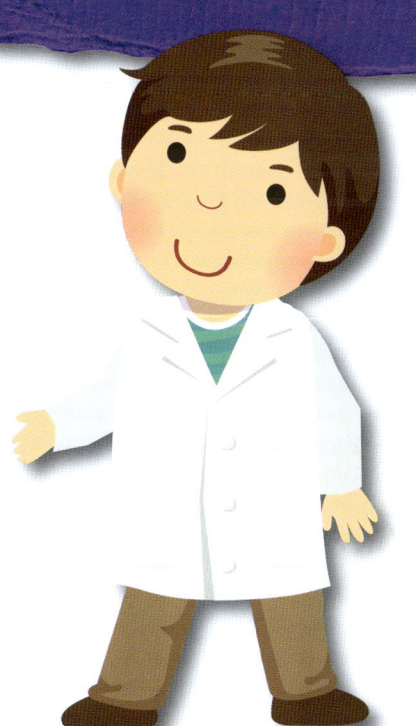

Today, we are visiting the dentist.

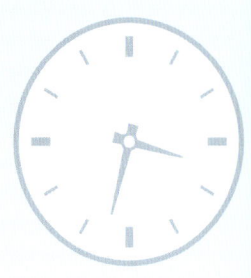

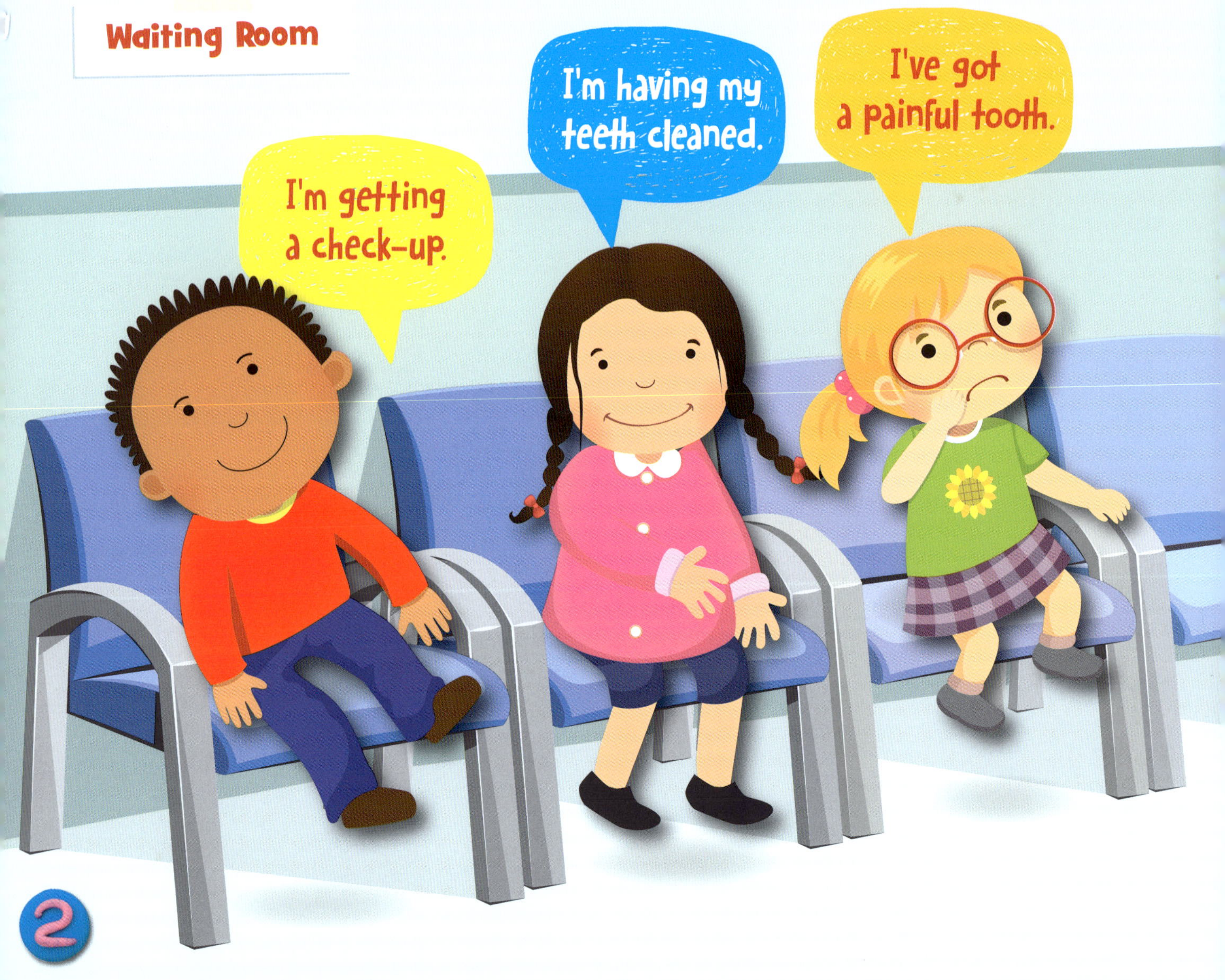

Waiting Room

I'm getting a check-up.

I'm having my teeth cleaned.

I've got a painful tooth.

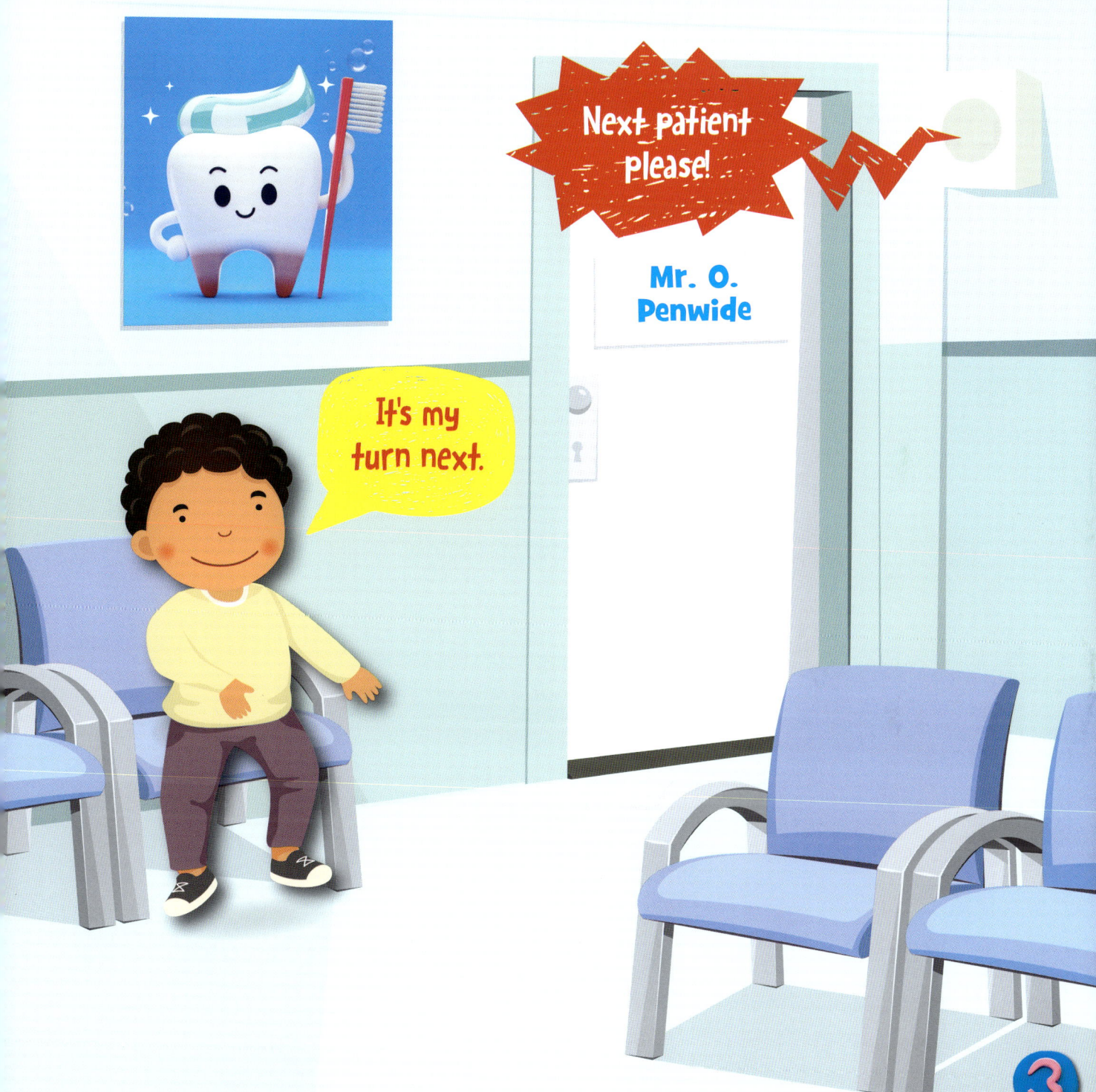

Dentists help people keep their teeth, gums and mouths healthy.

They have to learn lots of facts about teeth.

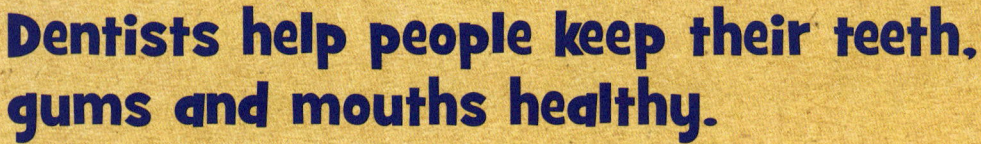

We have three main types of teeth.

Incisors cut food.

Canines tear food.

Molars grind food.

Teeth are covered in super hard enamel. Enamel is the hardest part of a person's body.

Dentists use SCIENCE to do their job.

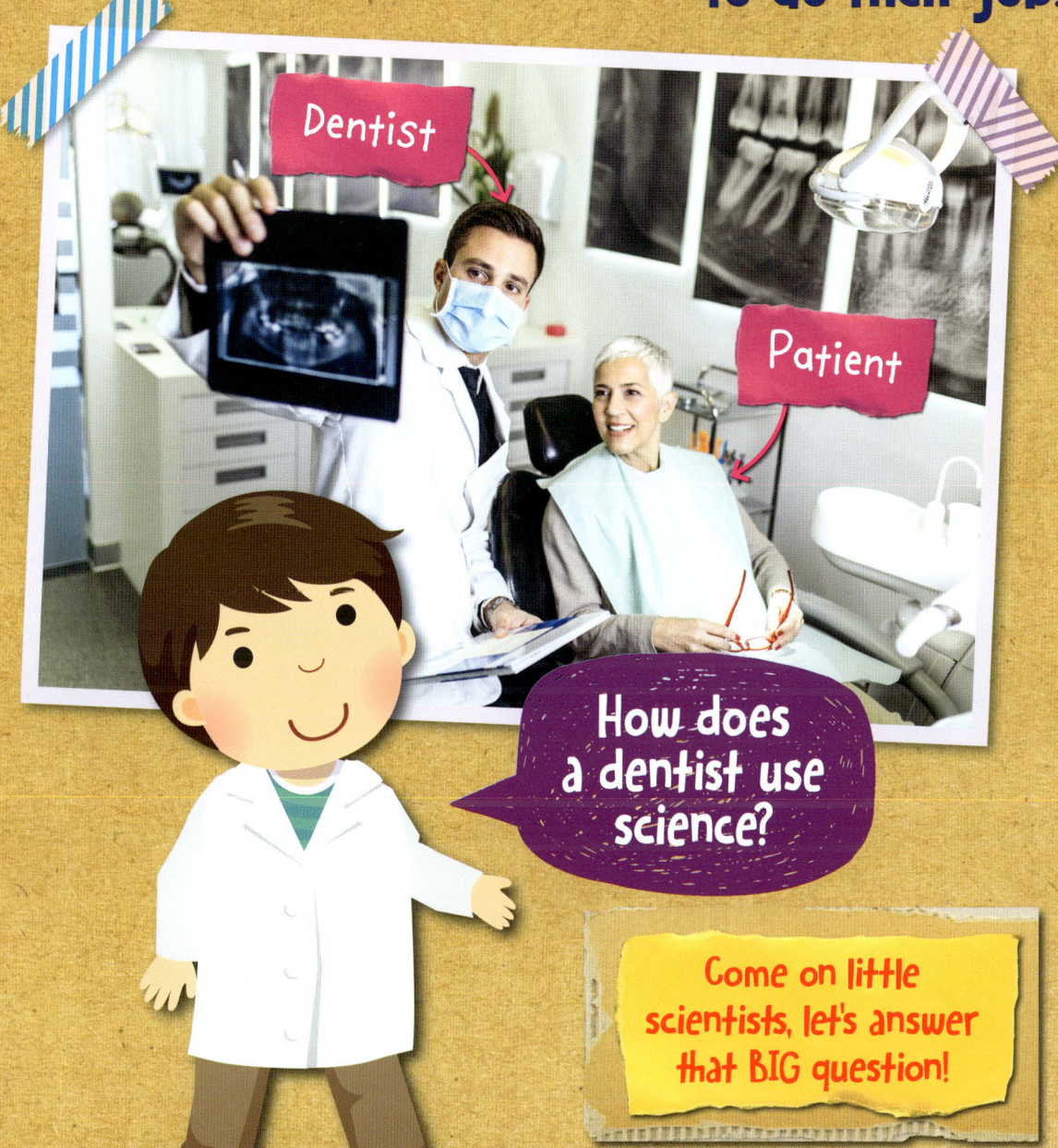

Dentist

Patient

How does a dentist use science?

Come on little scientists, let's answer that BIG question!

A dentist works in a room called a surgery.

The patient sits in a BIG chair.

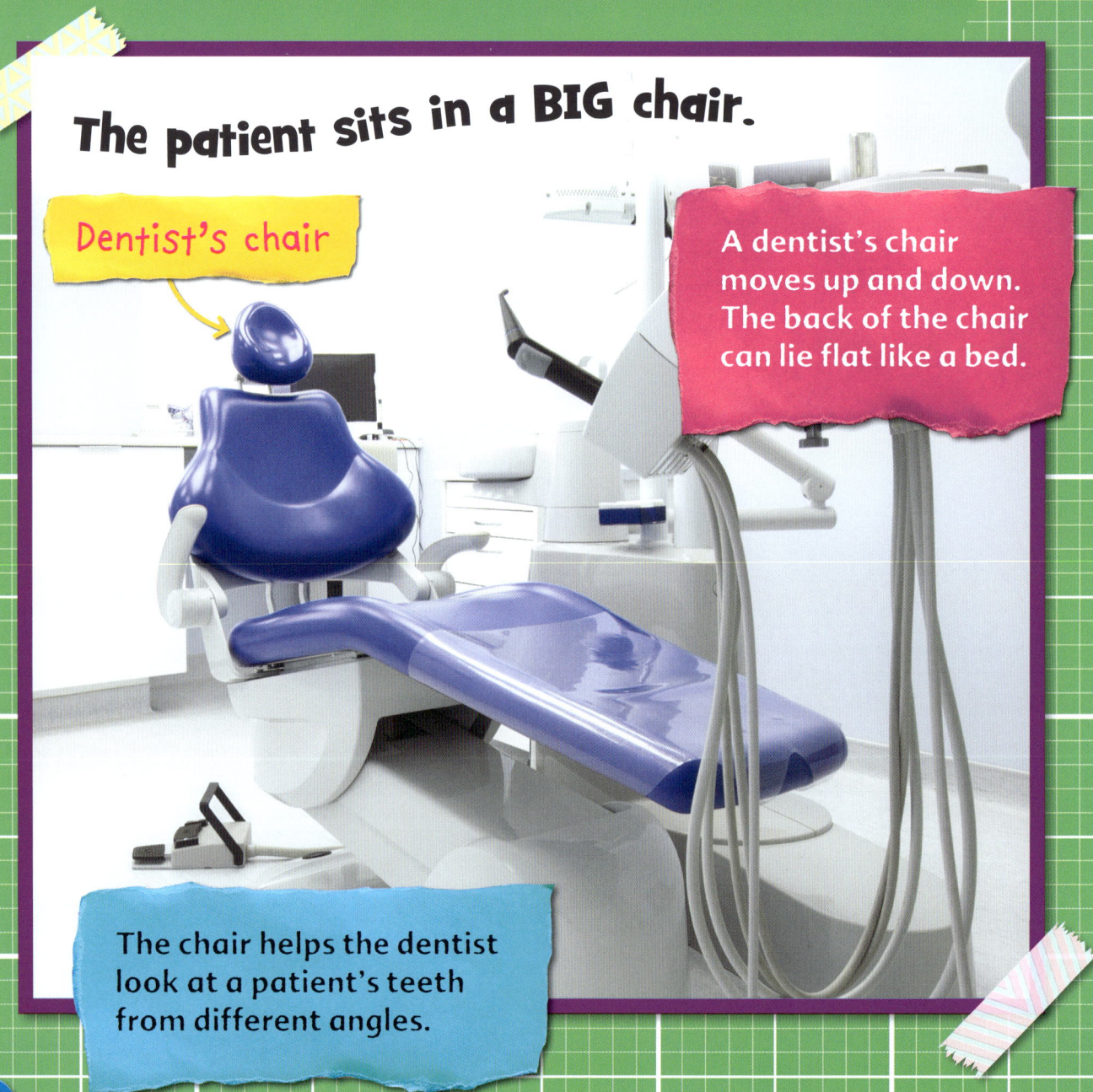

Dentist's chair

A dentist's chair moves up and down. The back of the chair can lie flat like a bed.

The chair helps the dentist look at a patient's teeth from different angles.

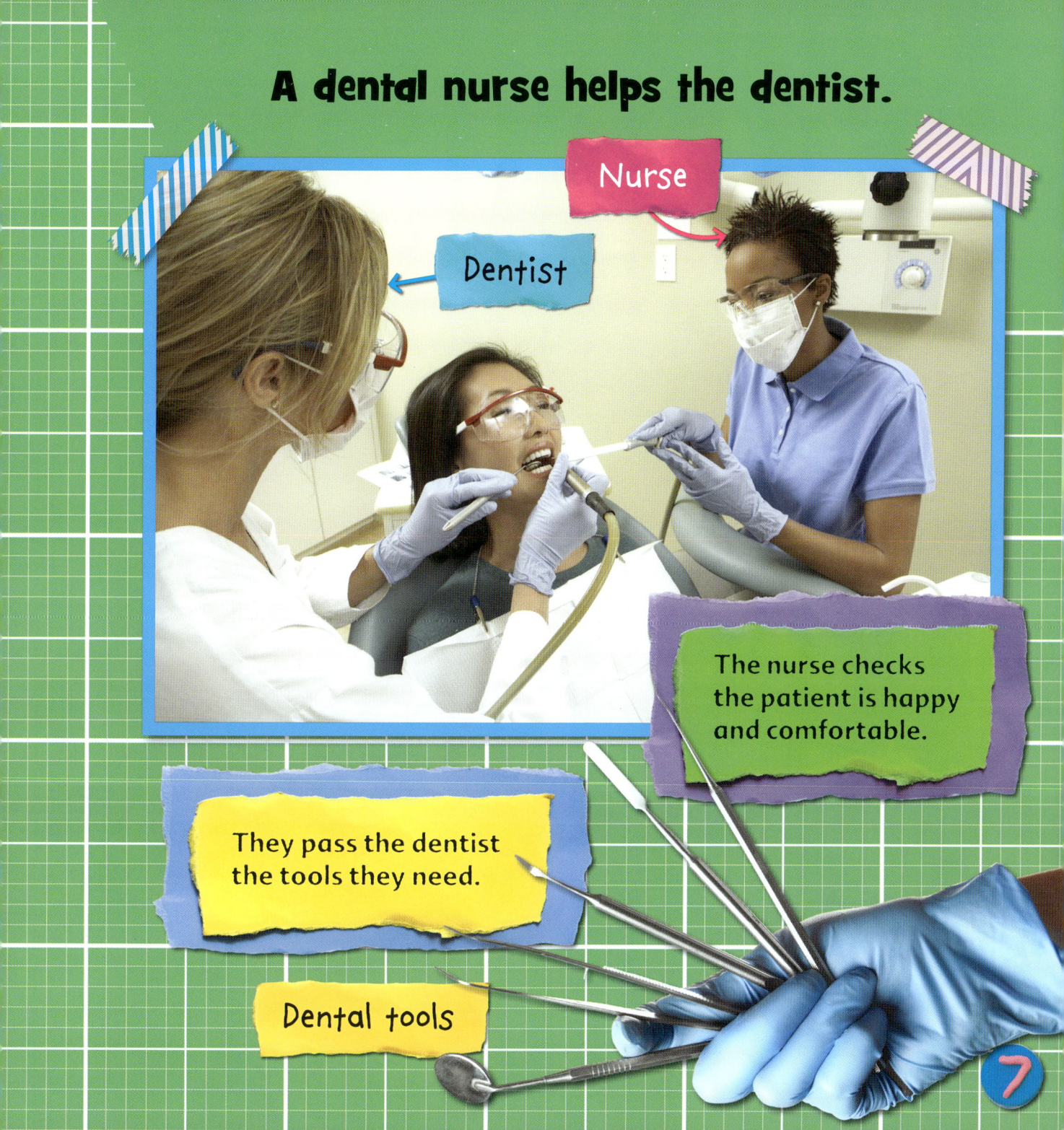

Time for a check-up!

The dentist shines a bright light in the patient's mouth to check the teeth.

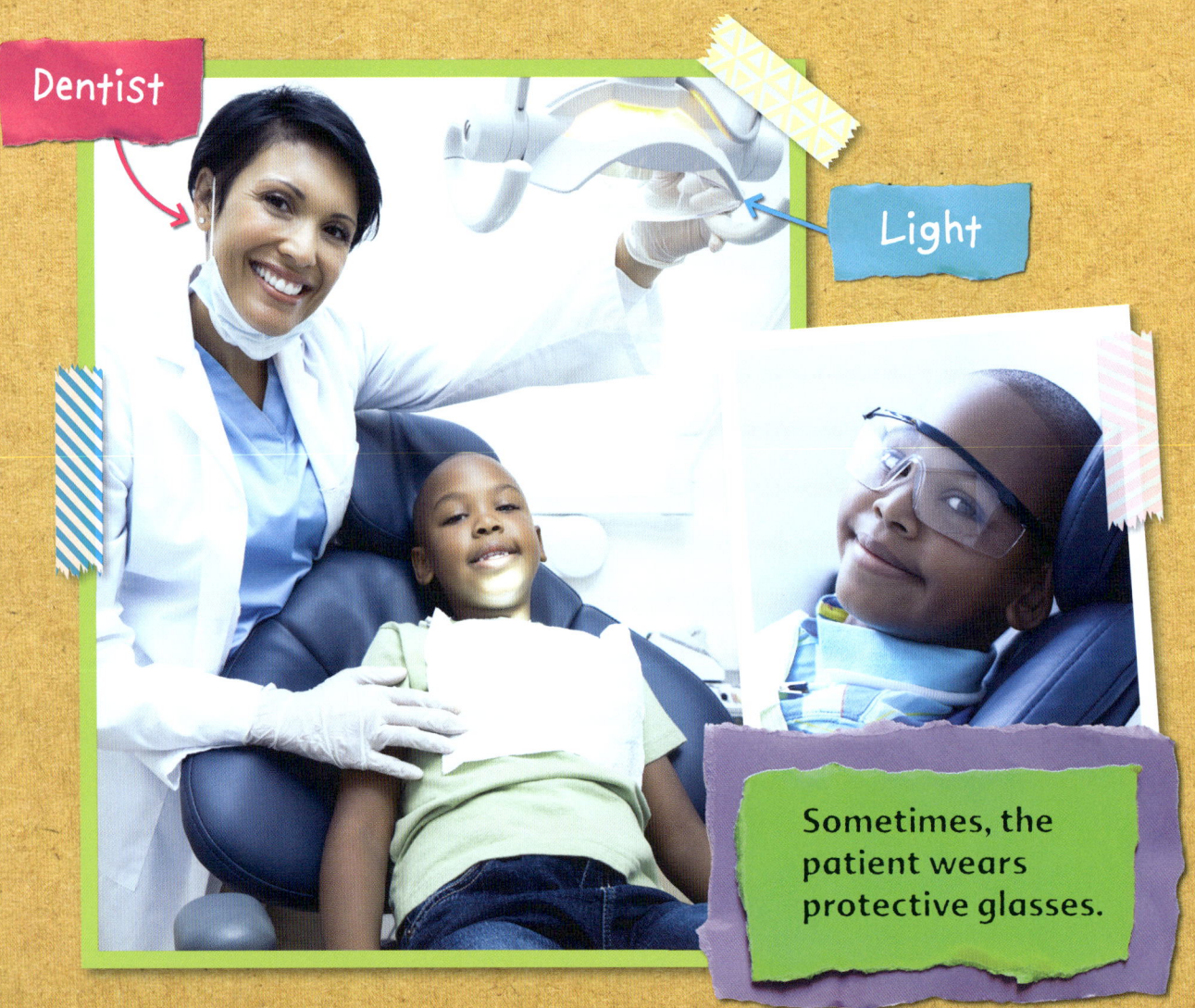

Dentist

Light

Sometimes, the patient wears protective glasses.

Our mouths are home to tiny living things called bacteria.

When bacteria and bits of food mix together, they make a sticky covering called plaque.

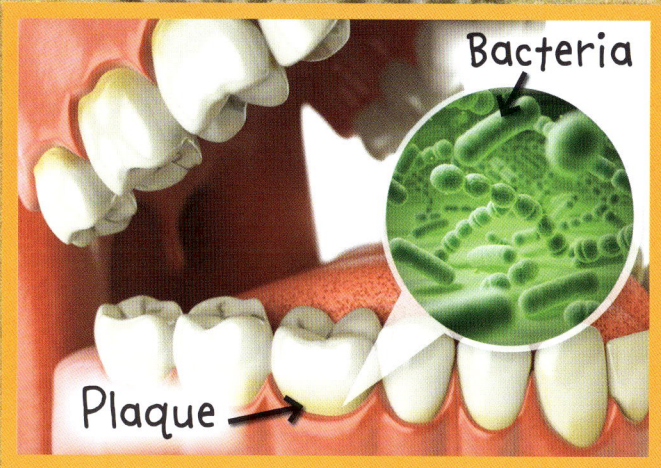

Plaque can damage your gums and cause tooth decay.

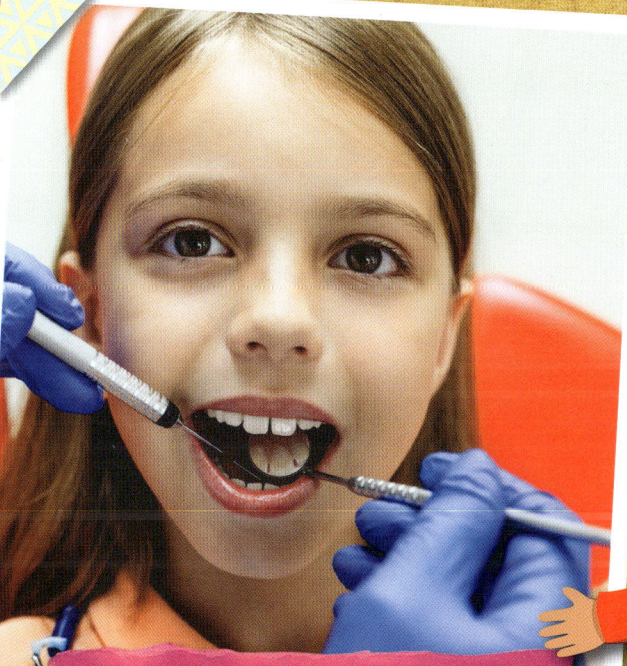

The dentist uses a mirror on a stick to look all around each tooth.

All done. My teeth and gums are healthy.

At the dentist, each tooth is given a number.

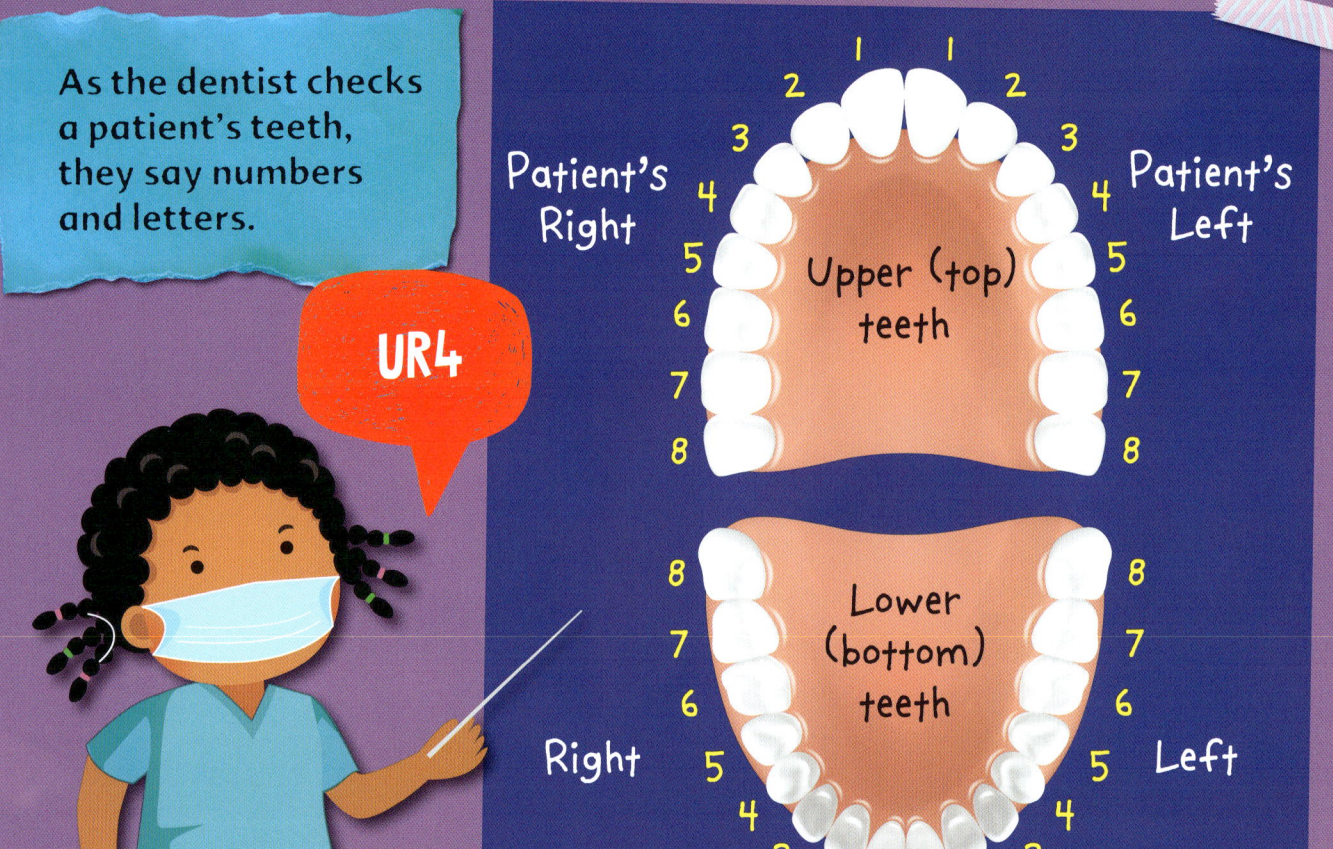

As the dentist checks a patient's teeth, they say numbers and letters.

UR4

UR4 means the dentist is talking about the Upper Right number 4 tooth.

The numbers and letters are like a dentist's code. They describe each tooth and its gum.

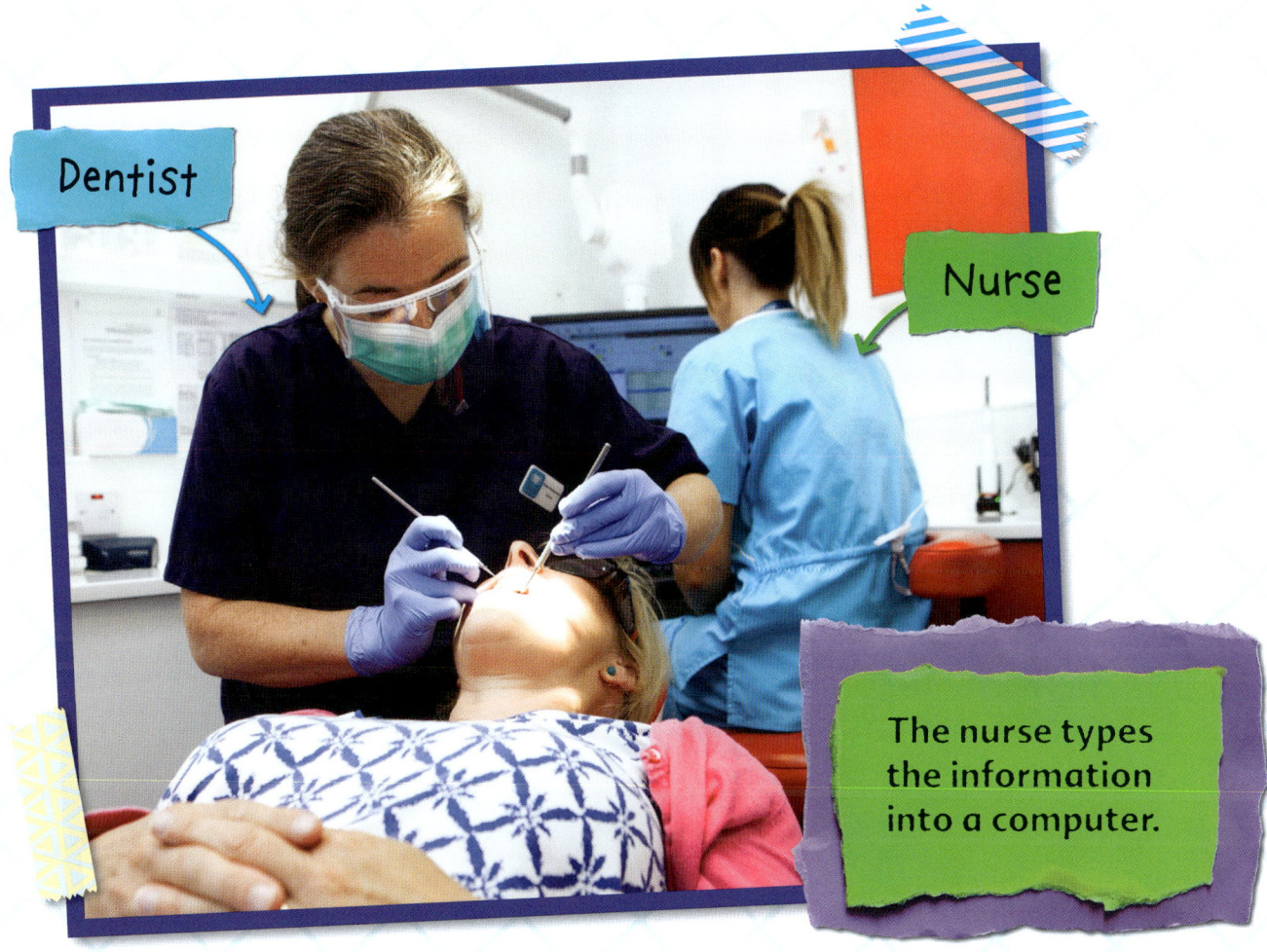

Dentist

Nurse

The nurse types the information into a computer.

The code helps the dentist keep a record of each tooth.

Sometimes a dentist uses an X-ray machine to take a picture of a person's teeth.

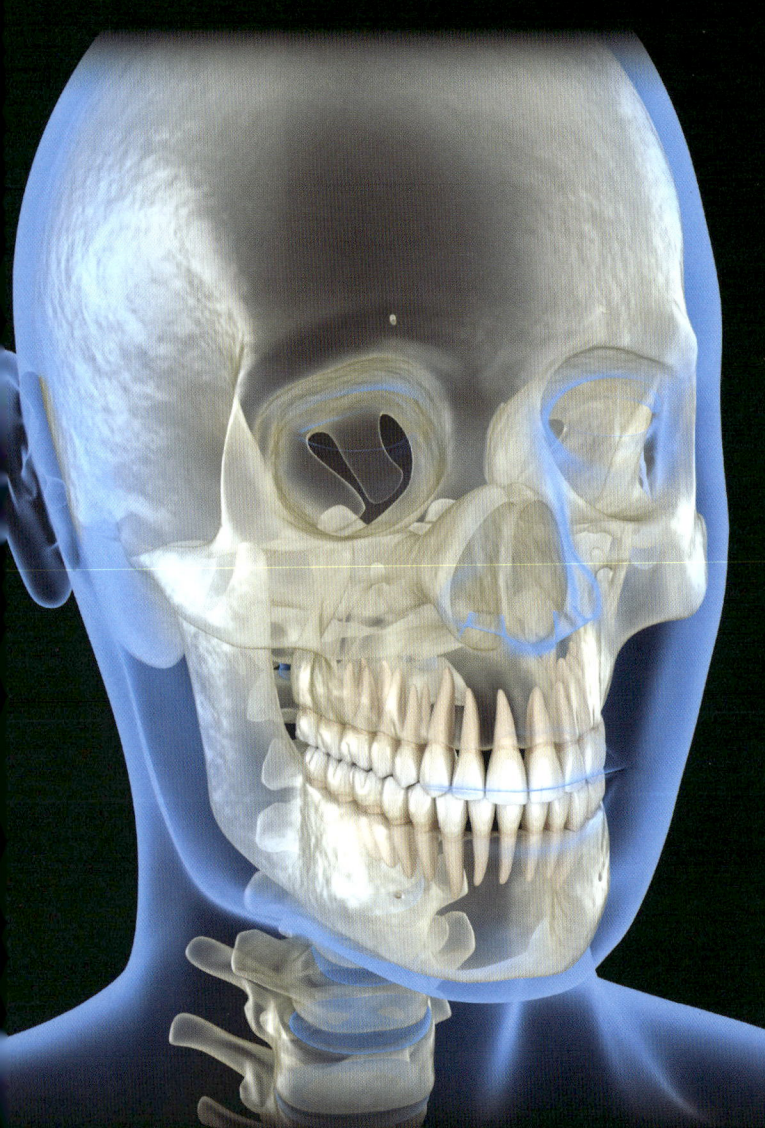

X-rays are pictures of what's inside a person's body.

Bones and teeth show up brightly on an X-ray picture.

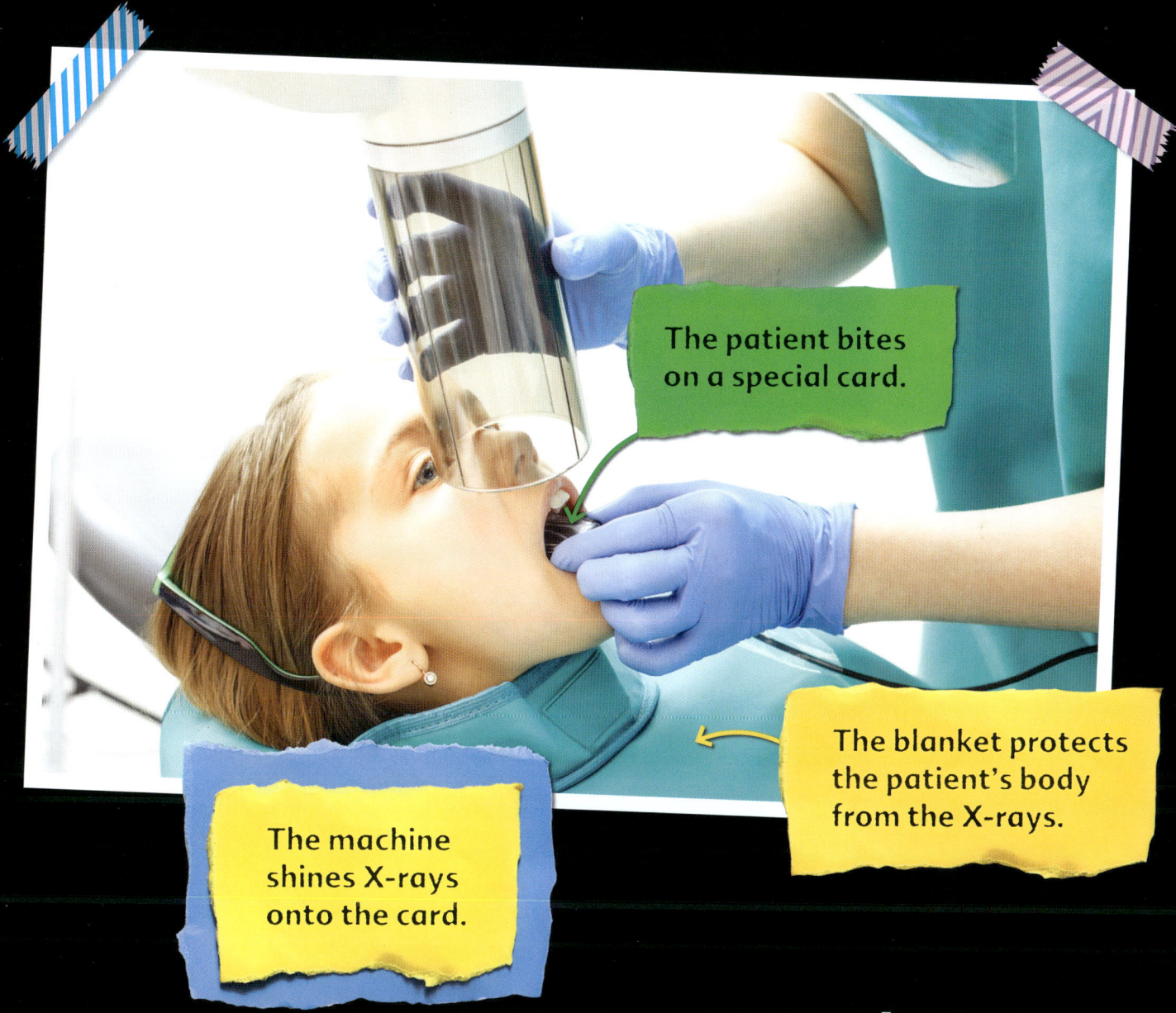

The patient bites on a special card.

The machine shines X-rays onto the card.

The blanket protects the patient's body from the X-rays.

X-rays can show problems in your bones, teeth and gums.

An X-ray can show that a patient has a small hole in their tooth. The hole is called a cavity and it can be painful.

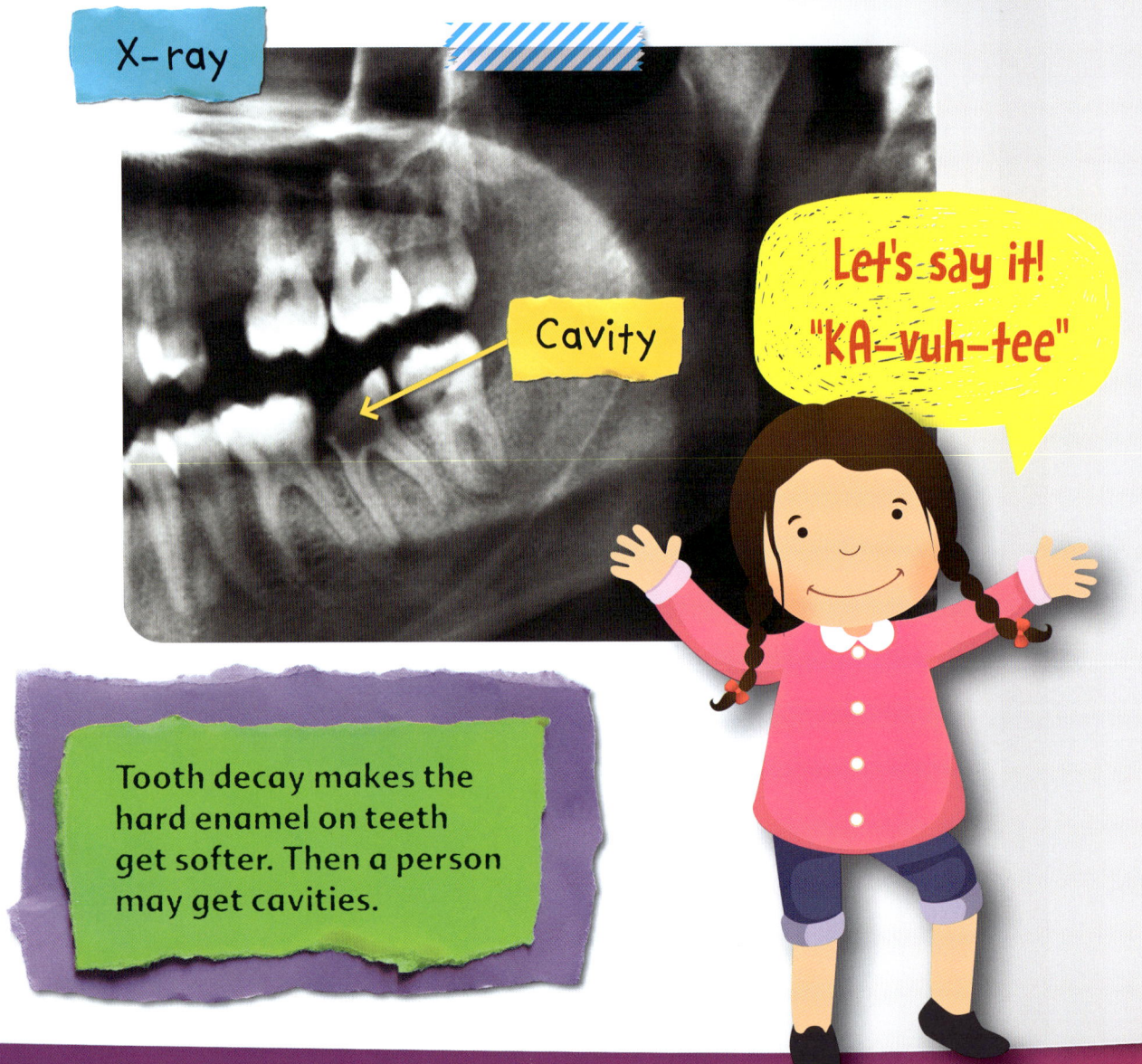

X-ray

Cavity

Let's say it! "KA-vuh-tee"

Tooth decay makes the hard enamel on teeth get softer. Then a person may get cavities.

A dentist uses science to fix a cavity.

First, the dentist gives the patient a special injection in their gums so they won't feel pain.

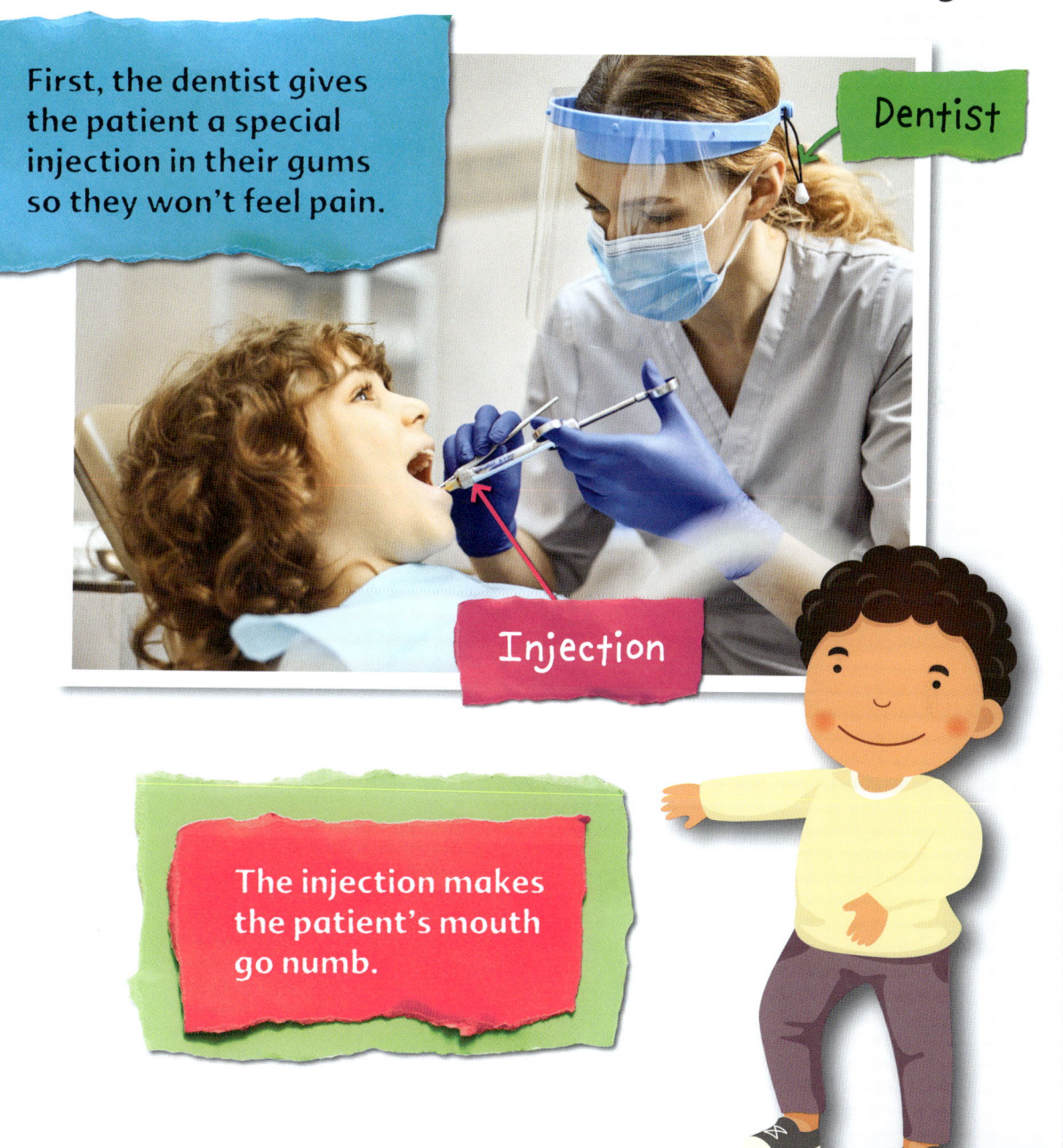

Dentist

Injection

The injection makes the patient's mouth go numb.

What happens next to fix a cavity?

The dentist uses a tiny drill to remove decaying, or bad, parts of the tooth around the cavity.

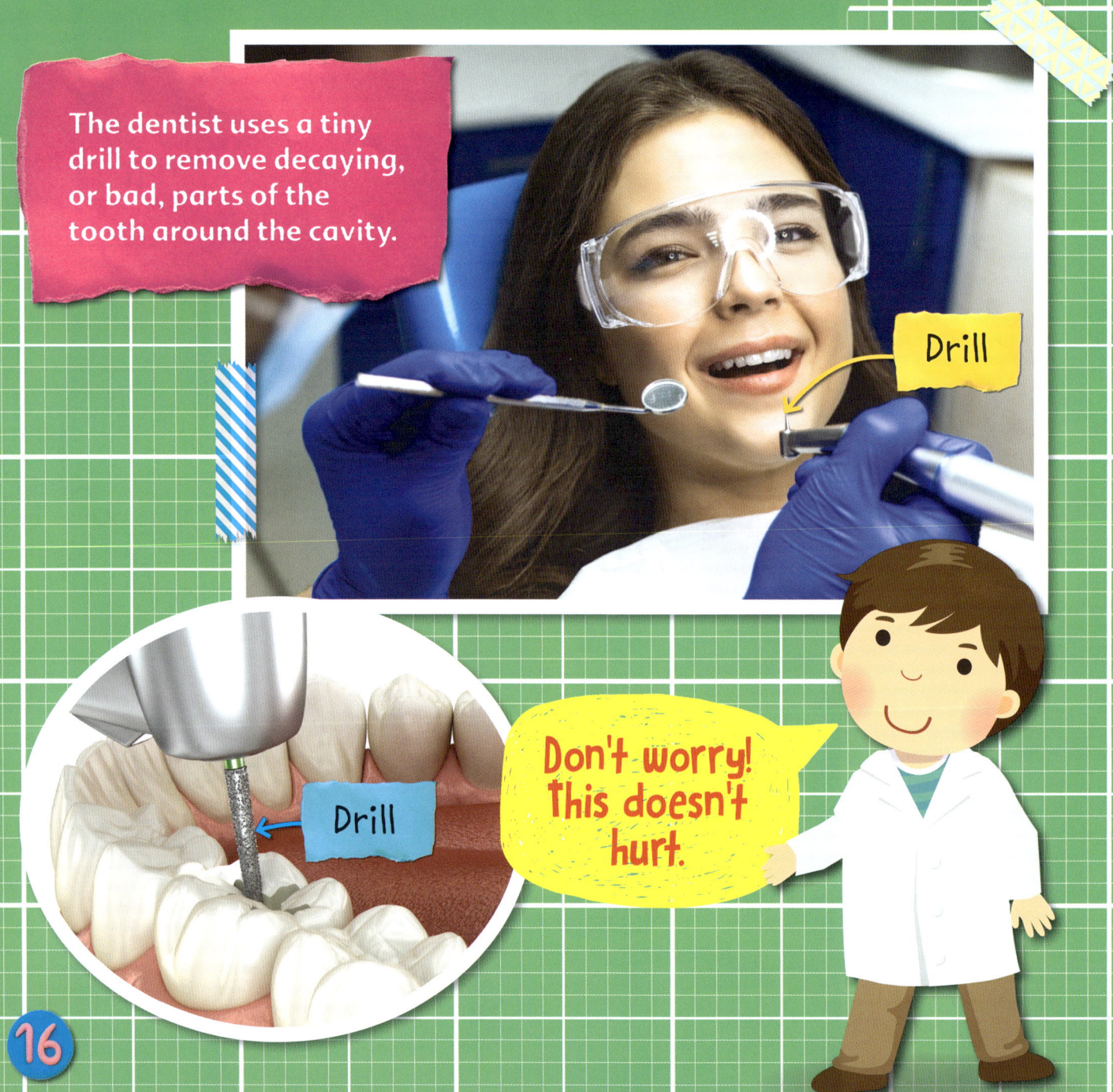

Drill

Drill

Don't worry! This doesn't hurt.

Then the dentist fills the hole with special tough material that goes hard.

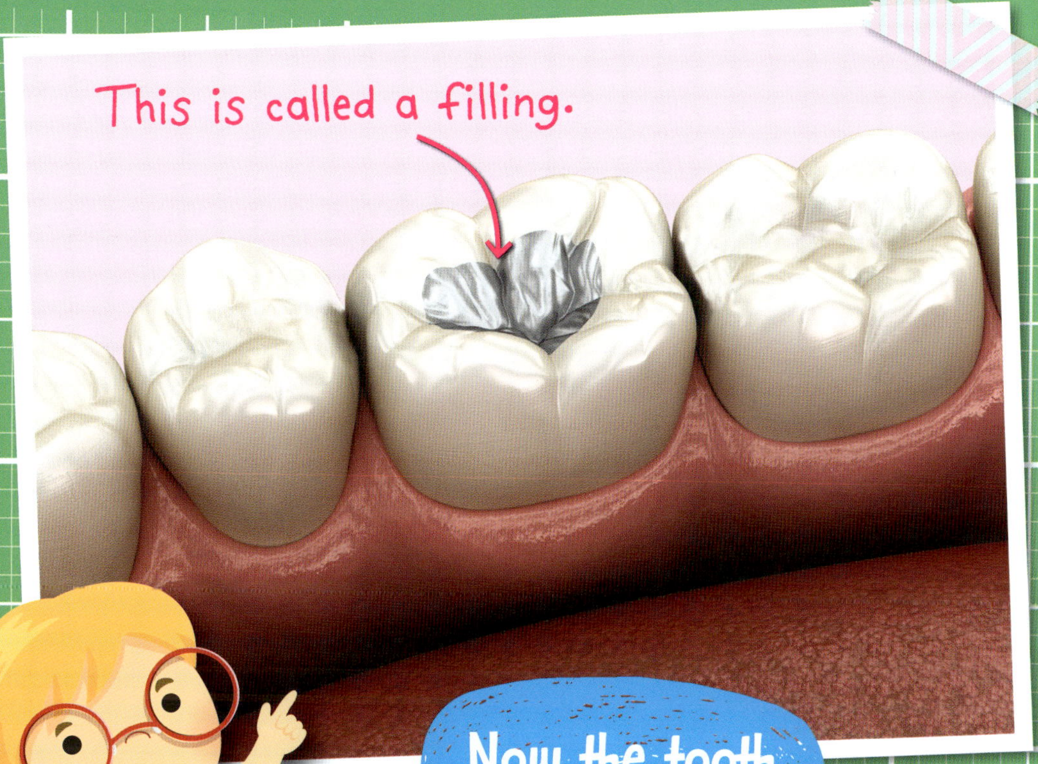

This is called a filling.

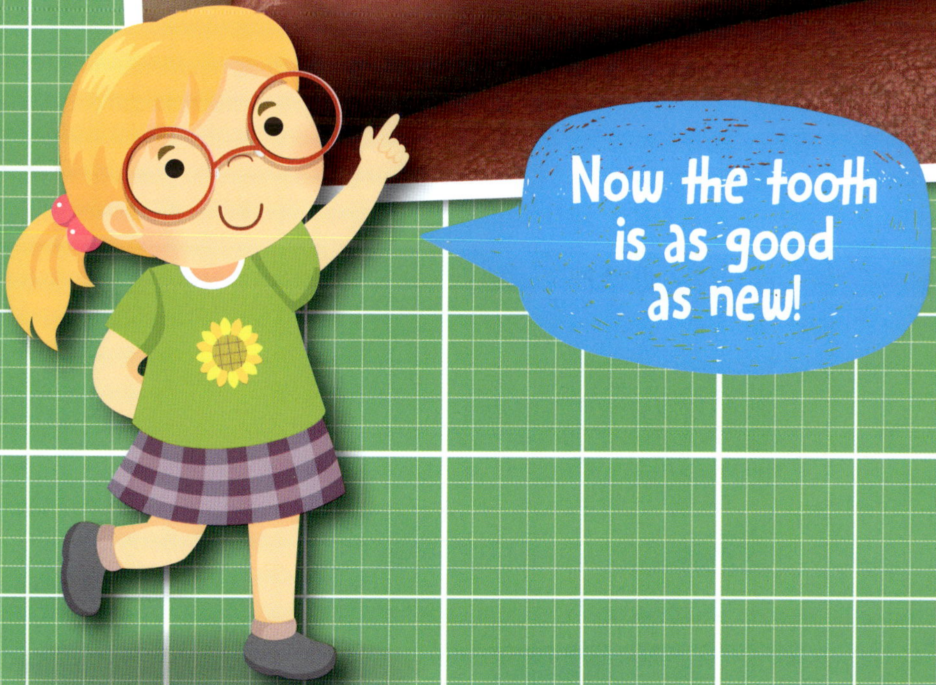

Now the tooth is as good as new!

A dentist can give a person's teeth a special clean.

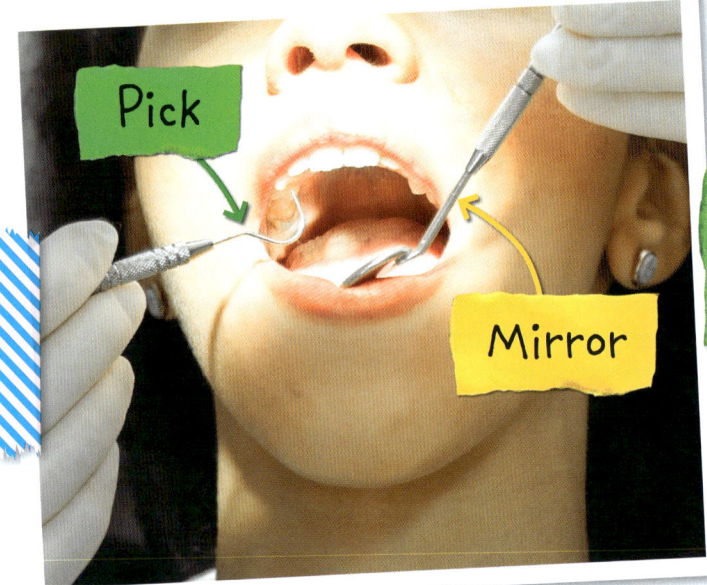

Pick

Mirror

Sometimes a tooth expert called a dental hygienist does this.

The dentist removes stuff called tartar with a tiny pick.

When plaque goes hard, it forms yellow tartar.

The dentist also removes plaque and tartar with an electric scaling tool.

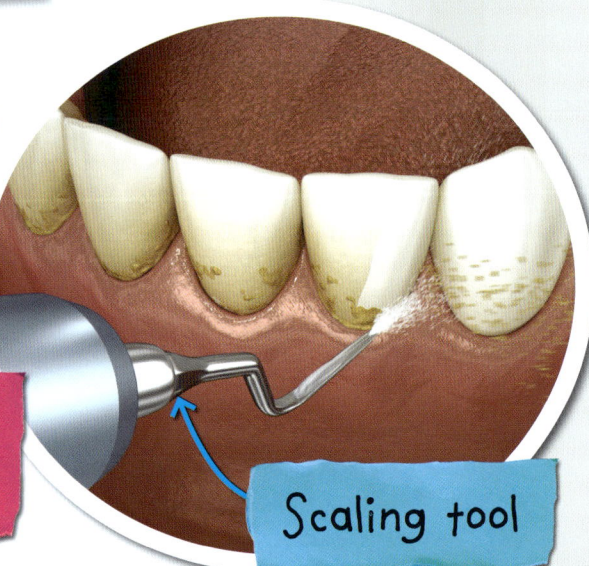

Water blasts from the tool.

Scaling tool

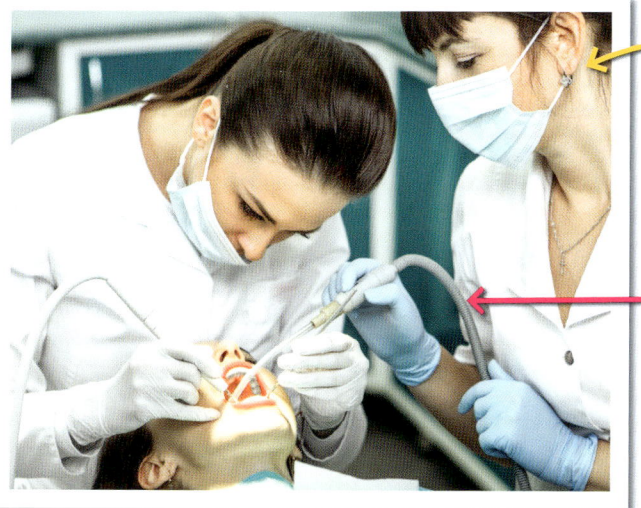

Nurse

This tube sucks up water and bits of tartar.

Finally, the dentist polishes the teeth.

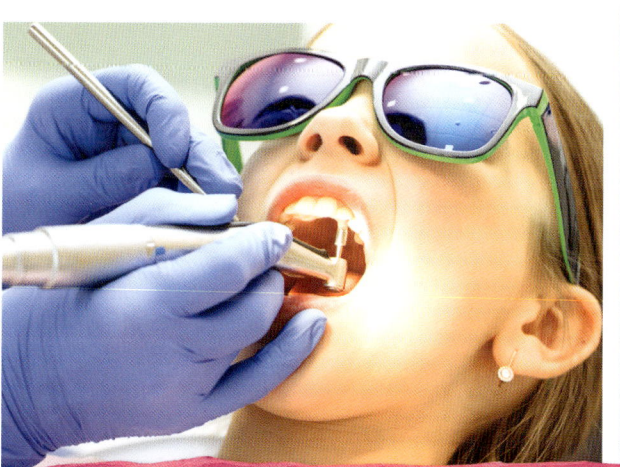

Now my teeth are smooth and shiny!

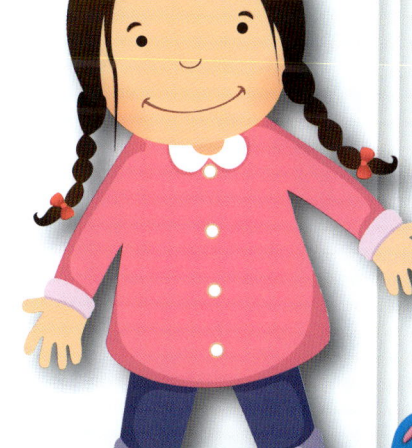

It's harder for plaque to stick to smooth, polished teeth.

Dentists teach us how to keep our teeth healthy.

Then we won't get toothache, tooth decay and cavities.

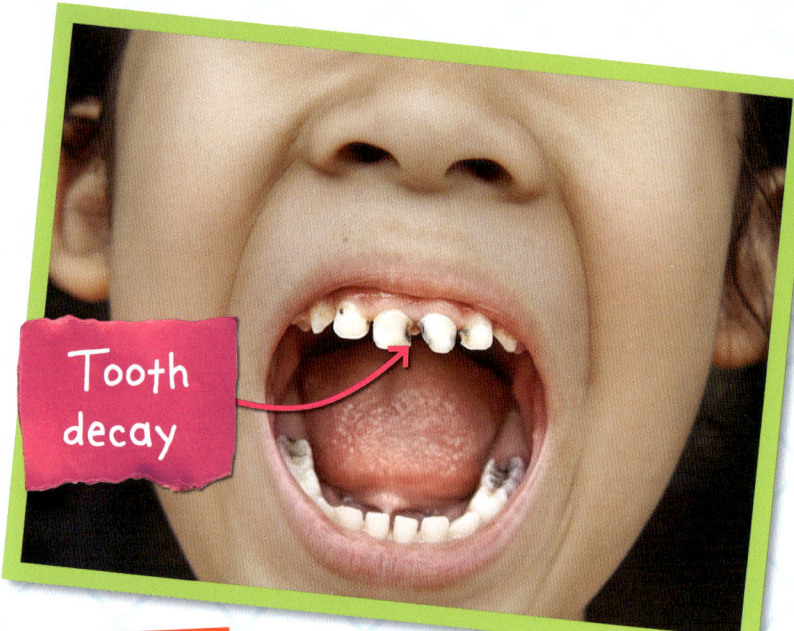

Tooth decay

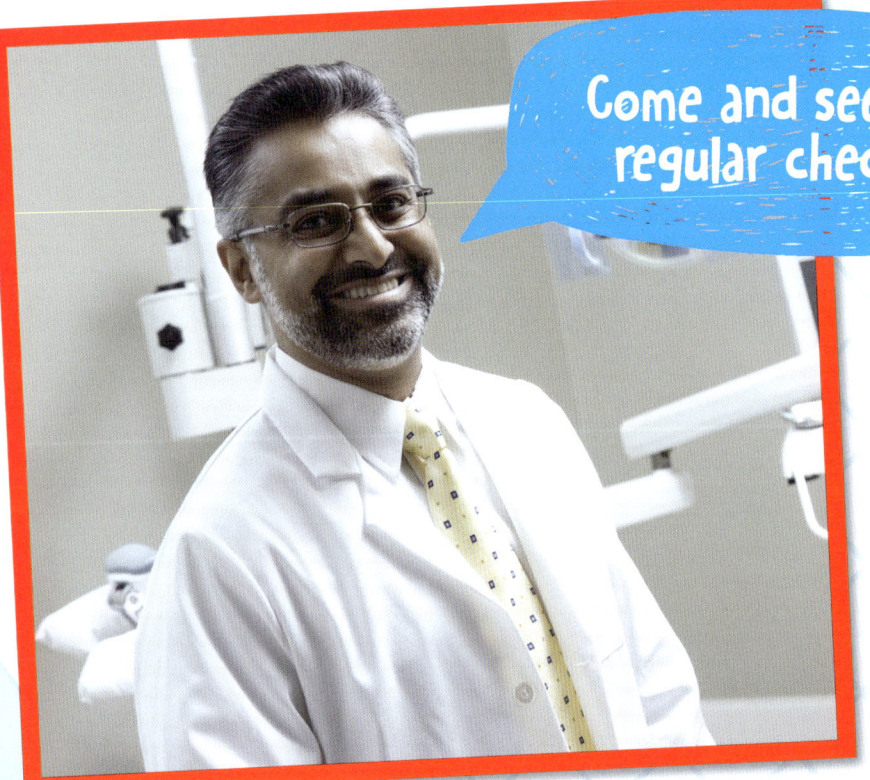

Come and see me for regular check-ups.

Don't drink sugary drinks.

Don't eat too many sugary sweets.

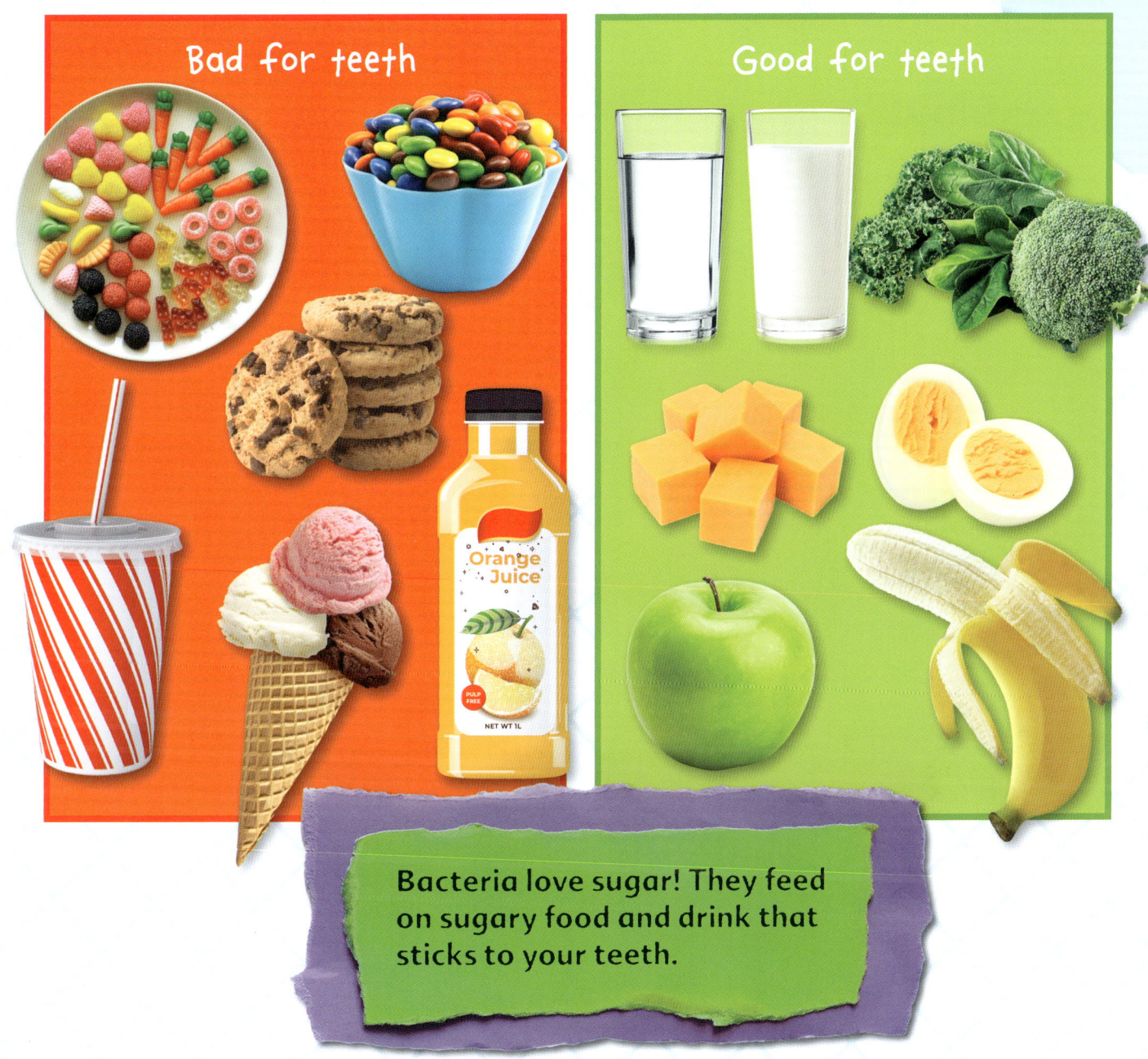

Bad for teeth

Good for teeth

Bacteria love sugar! They feed on sugary food and drink that sticks to your teeth.

That's why it's important to brush your teeth!

Brush your teeth twice every day for **2 minutes** each time.

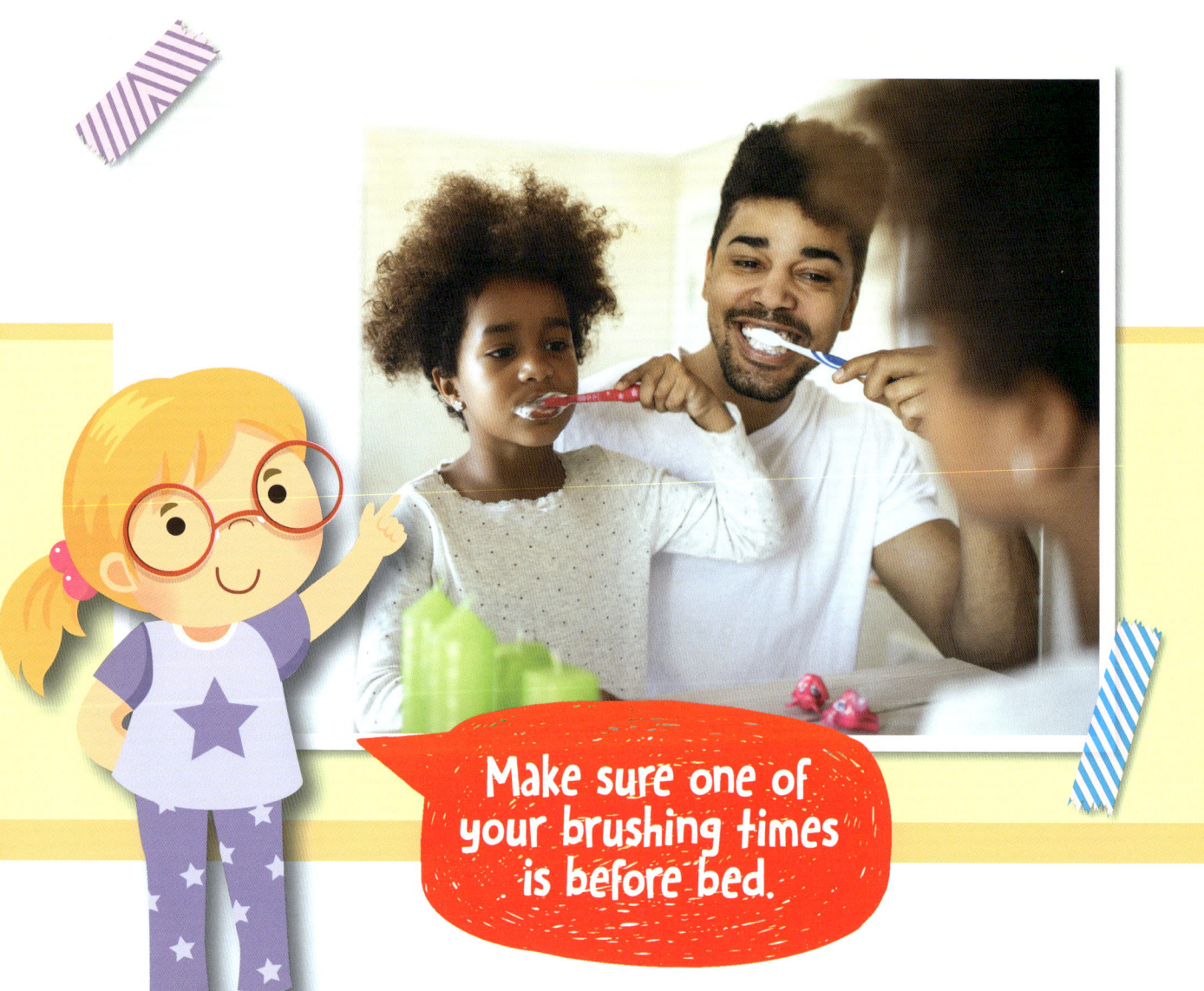

Make sure one of your brushing times is before bed.

There's a special stuff called fluoride that protects our teeth.

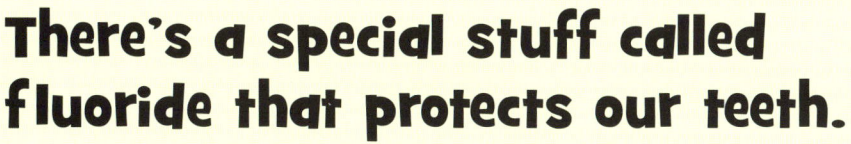

Scientists put fluoride in toothpaste. It helps strengthen the enamel on your teeth and stops tooth decay.

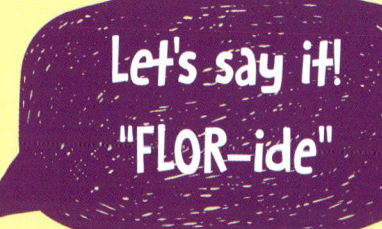

Let's say it! "FLOR-ide"

Now we know how dentists use science. Good work, little scientists!

My Science Words

cavity
A hole in a tooth that forms when a person has tooth decay.

enamel
The hard outer layer of your teeth.

plaque
A soft, sticky covering on teeth that is always forming. Brushing your teeth removes plaque.

tooth decay
Damage to your teeth that can make cavities and give you toothache. Decay happens when plaque mixes with sugary food and drinks in your mouth.

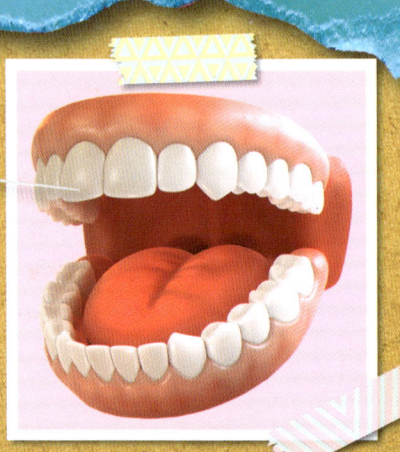